# Intermittent Fasting for Seniors

*An Essential Handbook for Vitality and Strength for Ageless Energy*

Healthy Happy Me

# Table of Contents

# Introduction

Retirement should have been a time of rest for Susan, but instead, it had become a time of worry and dismay. For years, Susan had been fighting a losing battle with her weight, and at the age of sixty-five, her health was in jeopardy. It seemed like no matter how hard she tried, she couldn't shed the extra pounds or keep them off. That is, until one day when Susan discovered the power of intermittent fasting.

This remarkable discovery changed her life and now Susan wants to share her story and help other seniors take control of their health and well-being. Intermittent fasting for seniors: "An Essential Handbook for Vitality and Strength for Ageless Energy."  is the perfect guide for those looking for a sustainable and effective way to lose weight and keep it off. From the basics of intermittent fasting to helpful tips and tricks, this comprehensive guide will provide you with the knowledge and advice to get started and achieve lasting success.

Let Susan show you how to take charge of your health and start living the life you deserve.

## Understanding the Power of Intermittent Fasting

## The Science Behind Ageless Energy

Fasting is purposely not eating food. In contrast, starvation is not being able to eat due to factors out of your control such as food security.

The origin of the practice of fasting dates back to ancient times when it was a common practice to fast to help heal the body. It also has roots in religion where it's said to help deepen your connection to your faith.

Intermittent fasting (IF) is gaining attention for its potential health benefits, particularly in weight management, blood pressure regulation, cholesterol reduction, diabetes prevention, and cognitive enhancement. This eating pattern involves alternating between fasting and eating periods, aiming to trigger fat-burning and promote metabolic efficiency.

Intermittent fasting can be done in various ways, there is no perfect fasting plan, it should be based on what works best in your life. If you don't eat for 10-16 hours, your body will go to its fat stores for energy, and fatty acids called ketones will be released into the bloodstream. This has been shown to protect memory and learning functionality. During meals, carbohydrates are broken down into glucose, which serves as the primary energy source for various bodily functions. Excess glucose is stored in the liver and adipose tissue as glycogen and fats, respectively. Between meals, when the body enters a fasted state, glycogen reserves are depleted, leading to the breakdown of fats into free fatty acids. These fatty acids are then converted into metabolic fuel in the liver, resulting in fat loss if the fasting period is prolonged.

Science Behind Intermittent Fasting



One key mechanism behind the benefits of intermittent fasting is its impact on insulin levels. Insulin, which facilitates glucose uptake by cells, is secreted in response to food intake. Constant high insulin levels, as seen with frequent eating throughout the day, can lead to insulin insensitivity, a precursor to type 2 diabetes. By keeping insulin levels low during fasting periods, intermittent fasting may help mitigate this risk.

Furthermore, intermittent fasting exerts positive effects on brain health by stimulating the production of neurotrophic factors, which support neuronal growth and survival. Similar to physical or cognitive exercise, fasting challenges the brain, potentially enhancing cognitive function and neuroplasticity.

While intermittent fasting shows promise, it may not be suitable for everyone. Individuals such as children, pregnant or breastfeeding women, those with eating disorders, type 1 diabetes, advanced diabetes, or certain medical conditions should avoid fasting. Additionally, fasting should be approached with caution and done correctly to prevent potential risks.

One of the simplest intermittent fasting methods involves extending the nighttime fast, typically with a 16-hour fasting period followed by an 8-hour eating window. It is essential to maintain balanced nutrition during eating periods and stay hydrated while fasting. Breaking the fast gradually and avoiding overeating, especially unhealthy foods, is crucial for safety and effectiveness.

One method is fasting daily for a set amount of time, usually 12 hours or more. The average person sleeps about 7 hours a night, which counts towards that fasting time. If you don't eat after dinner, then you could easily achieve a daily fast to help your body burn fat more efficiently. This type of fasting can help night snackers. Intermittent fasting is not about eating heaps of high-calorie, high-fat foods, such as hamburgers, French fries, and cakes. The implication is that if you fast two days a week, you can devour as much junk as your gullet can swallow during the remaining five days. Some studies propose eating sensibly most of the time, eating nothing for an extended period now and then, indulge only on occasion (perhaps once a week, say on a designated "cheat day")

## Benefits for Seniors

Intermittent fasting holds significant potential for improving the health and well-being of seniors, offering a range of benefits tailored to their specific needs and concerns.

**1. Improves Biomarkers of Disease:** For seniors, maintaining optimal health becomes increasingly crucial. Intermittent fasting has been shown to improve various biomarkers of disease, such as reducing inflammation, blood sugar levels, and cholesterol levels. These improvements can contribute to a lower risk of chronic diseases commonly associated with aging, such as cardiovascular disease, diabetes, and neurodegenerative disorders.

**2. Reduces Oxidative Stress:** Oxidative stress, resulting from an imbalance between free radicals and antioxidants in the body, plays a significant role in aging and age-related diseases. Intermittent fasting has been found to reduce oxidative stress by enhancing the body's antioxidant defenses. This can help protect seniors' cells and tissues from damage, potentially slowing down the aging process and reducing the risk of age-related conditions.

**3. Preserve Learning and Memory Functioning:**
Cognitive decline is a common concern among seniors,
but intermittent fasting may offer a protective effect on
brain health. Studies suggest that intermittent fasting can
preserve learning and memory functioning by promoting
neuroplasticity and increasing the production of
neurotrophic factors, which support the growth and
survival of neurons. By maintaining cognitive function,
intermittent fasting may help seniors maintain
independence and quality of life as they age.

**4. Psychological Benefits:** Fasting periods induce a mild
stress response in cells, triggering adaptive mechanisms
that enhance resilience and resistance to disease. This
adaptive stress response may extend beyond the physical
benefits of fasting to include psychological benefits.
Seniors may experience improved mood, mental clarity,
and overall psychological well-being during fasting
periods. Additionally, the sense of accomplishment and
discipline associated with intermittent fasting can
contribute to a positive mindset and sense of control over

one's                                        health.

# Chapter One

## Getting Started

### Preparing for a Successful Journey

Susan's experience with weight and health predates her decision to follow an intermittent fasting regimen. She is reminded of her mother's ongoing battle with dieting when she thinks back to her adolescent years. Her mother, a dance instructor by trade, represented the social pressure placed on women to uphold a particular physical appearance. Growing up in this milieu, Susan couldn't escape the prevailing assumption that being slim was synonymous with success and pleasure.

She first became aware of dieting during her first year of college when she discovered she had gained the dreaded "freshman 15." And so began a wild trip filled with diets and weight swings. Like so many others, Susan was consumed with trying every diet that claimed to provide a quick remedy for her weight problems. She made an effort, but success eluded her, and she was left in a never-ending cycle of hope and despair.

Around 2009, Susan became aware of intermittent fasting for the first time, but she didn't fully commit to incorporating it into her life until 2014. She went through years of ups and downs before a family vacation made her face the harsh truth of her weight gain. Susan became aware that she was technically obese when her weight reached 210 pounds, and she knew she needed to change.

Susan decided to give intermittent fasting a serious try during this moment of clarity. She lost eighty pounds and kept it off through menopause with hard work and determination. She credits her success to realizing the value of clean fasting and accepting intermittent fasting as a way of life rather than just a diet.

To provide you with the knowledge and inspiration to embark on this transformative path toward better health and well-being, we'll explore Susan's experiences and insights in this chapter. We'll also dispel many myths and misconceptions about intermittent fasting so that you have a clear understanding of what it involves. So let's get started on this journey together, knowing that we can achieve lasting success with perseverance and the right guidance.

## Common Myths and Misconceptions about Intermittent Fasting for Seniors

### Myth #1: Fasting Slows Down Your Metabolism

One of the most pervasive myths surrounding intermittent fasting is the belief that it slows down metabolism, sabotaging weight loss efforts. This misconception often stems from concerns about the body entering "starvation mode," where metabolic processes grind to a halt, making it harder to burn fat.

Contrary to this belief, research suggests that short-term fasting can enhance metabolism. When you fast, your body undergoes a metabolic shift, transitioning from burning carbohydrates to utilizing stored fat for fuel.

This transition is accompanied by an increase in norepinephrine, a hormone that stimulates metabolism and accelerates fat breakdown.

Moreover, intermittent fasting has been shown to improve metabolic health over time, potentially reducing the risk of digestive disorders. Therefore, rather than impeding metabolism, fasting may enhance its function, promoting efficient fat-burning and metabolic regulation.

**Myth #2: Fasting Makes You Lose Muscle**

Another prevalent myth is the fear that fasting leads to muscle loss, which can undermine efforts to build or maintain strength. Some individuals worry that reducing meal frequency may limit the body's ability to support muscle development, resulting in decreased muscle mass.

However, research suggests that fasting can preserve lean muscle mass and, in some cases, stimulate muscle growth. During fasting periods, the body increases the production of growth hormones necessary for muscle building and preservation.

It's important to note that muscle loss during fasting is typically associated with inadequate protein intake or extreme fasting methods. By ensuring a balanced diet rich in protein and engaging in strength training exercises, seniors can mitigate the risk of muscle loss while fasting.

**Myth #3: Fasting Causes Nutrient Deficiencies**

There is a common misconception that fasting leads to nutrient deficiencies due to reduced calorie intake. However, when practiced sensibly, fasting may positively impact nutrient absorption and utilization.

Fasting provides valuable periods of rest for the digestive system, allowing it to function more efficiently and improve nutrient absorption. Additionally, fasting can promote better eating habits and encourage the consumption of nutrient-dense foods during eating windows.

While fasting may pose a risk of nutrient deficiencies if not properly planned, this can be mitigated by following a balanced diet and incorporating a variety of vitamins and minerals-rich foods into meals.

**Myth #4: Fasting is Unsafe**

Fasting has often been criticized as an unsafe and unhealthy practice, especially among seniors concerned about dehydration and disruptions to bodily functions. However, when practiced responsibly, fasting is safe and offers several health benefits.

To ensure safe fasting, it's essential to prioritize hydration and consult with healthcare professionals before embarking on a fasting regimen, especially for seniors with certain medical conditions. By adopting a mindful approach to fasting and adhering to safety guidelines, seniors can harness its potential benefits while minimizing potential risks.

These common myths underscore the importance of seeking accurate information and approaching intermittent fasting with mindfulness and moderation. By dispelling these misconceptions, seniors can make informed decisions about incorporating intermittent fasting into their lifestyle to promote overall health and well-being.

# Chapter Two

# The Golden Hours Approach

## Exploring the Concept of Ageless Energy

Sundays and special events were revered times of family bonding and wisdom-sharing when I was a child growing up in a small Dominican community. Our home-grown food served as more than just nourishment; it was a link between generations. One lesson that has stuck with me over the years is from my grandma, the matriarch of our family. She put her own needs first, understanding that taking care of herself was the cornerstone of her ability to take care of the whole family. Her insight embodied a respect for the elderly, realizing their crucial role in the health of our community.

The story changes amid the busy streets of New York City. Even if they are many in number, the elderly frequently disappear into the turmoil of the city. Nonetheless, they undoubtedly make up a sizable portion of the city's population. The preoccupation with anti-aging products stems from a widespread fear of aging in society. I disagree with this viewpoint, viewing aging's beauty as a blessing and a mark of a life well spent.

Rather than being a hindrance to life, age is a doorway to renewed vigor. We need to recognize that the retirement experience is changing as the baby boomer generation does. Although longevity presents many chances for development and involvement, it also necessitates a change in how we handle elder care.

## Tailoring Intermittent Fasting to Senior Lifestyles

Intermittent fasting, which is customized to fit the distinct lives of seniors, is one of the most effective strategies in this paradigm shift. Traditional concepts of fasting may seem frightening or impossible for older folks, but with intelligent adaption, it can become a cornerstone           of          ageless           vigor.

Intermittent fasting is not only about limitation; it is a balanced approach to sustenance and renewal. Seniors can maximize their energy levels, cognitive performance, and general well-being by carefully planning their meals and incorporating fasting times. However, this technique needs to be sensitive to the unique demands and difficulties older individuals confront.

For people with a marginal body weight, there is an increased concern of a more significant weight loss which can affect the bones, overall immune system, and energy level. People who need to take their medications with food to avoid nausea or stomach irritation may not do well with fasting. Also, people who take heart or blood pressure medications may be more likely to suffer dangerous imbalances in Potassium and Sodium when they're fasting. Intermittent fasting may also be harmful if you have diabetes and need food at certain times or take medication that affects your blood sugar.

## Strategies for Tailoring Senior's Lifestyle to Fit Intermittent Fasting Regime

1. **Select an appropriate fasting technique:** Instead of extending your fasts, seniors may choose less stringent techniques like time-restricted eating, in which they fast for a shorter period each day (such as 12–14 hours). By doing this, the chance of both extreme weight loss and nutrient deficits can be reduced.

2. **Keep an eye on hydration and nutritional intake**: To maintain general health and avoid deficiencies, seniors should make sure they are getting enough water and nutrients throughout mealtimes. To assist meet nutritional needs, including nutrient-dense foods including fruits, vegetables, lean meats, and whole grains.

3. **Modify fasting schedule**: Seniors may need to modify their fasting regimen to account for medical issues or prescription needs. It is essential for safety to work with a healthcare provider to create a fasting schedule that fits in with prescription regimens and blood sugar control.

4. **Closely check health:** When engaging in intermittent fasting, seniors should keep a constant eye on their health and well-being. It can be helpful to monitor energy levels, mood, cognitive function, and general physical health to detect any negative effects and modify the fasting schedule as needed.

5. **Take into account alternate dietary approaches:** Seniors should investigate alternate dietary approaches that support health and well-being if intermittent fasting is not appropriate or presents hazards for specific medical conditions. Balanced meal planning, portion control, and regular exercise are a few examples of this.

6. **Put safety and well-being first:** When thinking about intermittent fasting or making any dietary adjustments,

seniors should put their safety and well-being first. A healthy and long-lasting approach to fasting can be ensured by being aware of specific health demands and making well-informed selections after consulting with healthcare                                              professionals.

Seniors can adapt their lifestyle to intermittent fasting in a way that supports safety, well-being, and health by following these guidelines and consulting with medical specialists                                              frequently

# Chapter Three

# Essential Guidelines

It is important to note that before you embark on the journey of intermittent fasting as a senior follow the appropriate guidelines to ensure your journey goes smoothly. There are various types of intermittent fasting, all of which will be explained in detail in this chapter. It does not matter which intermittent fasting approach you follow just ensuring that it suits your basic lifestyle needs makes it an ideal choice.

## Types of Intermittent Fasting

**1. Alternate Day Fasting(ADF)**

Alternate-day fasting (ADF) is a form of intermittent fasting where individuals alternate between fasting and normal eating days. ADF involves fasting on one day and then eating normally on the next. Some variants allow around 500 calories on fasting days, making it more sustainable for many individuals. Beverages like water, unsweetened coffee, and tea are permitted on fasting days.

**Weight Loss:**

While ADF may aid weight loss, studies suggest it's not significantly more effective than traditional daily calorie restriction. ADF can help reduce body weight and fat mass, with comparable results to other calorie-restricted diets. Combining ADF with exercise may enhance weight loss.

**Hunger:**

The effects of ADF on hunger are inconsistent, with some experiencing reduced hunger over time. Modified ADF with 500 calories on fasting days is generally more tolerable than full fasts. Compensatory hunger, common in continuous calorie restriction, doesn't seem to increase with ADF.

**Body Composition:**

ADF may help preserve lean muscle mass during weight loss, although recent evidence suggests it's no more effective than other calorie restriction methods.

**Health Benefits:**

ADF offers various health benefits, including reducing risk factors for type 2 diabetes and improving heart health. It may decrease fasting insulin levels and lower blood pressure, LDL cholesterol, and triglycerides.

**Autophagy:**

ADF stimulates autophagy, a cellular process linked to disease prevention and longevity. However, further research is needed to fully understand its effects on autophagy and longevity in humans.

**Safety:**

ADF is generally safe for most individuals but may not be suitable for certain populations like children, pregnant or lactating women, or those with specific medical conditions. Consulting a healthcare provider before starting ADF is recommended.

## 2. Eat Stop Eat

Eat Stop Eat is an intermittent fasting method that entails two days of 24-hour fasting per week, interspersed with five days of regular eating. It's characterized by flexibility and simplicity, allowing you to choose your fasting days and eat as you wish on non-fasting days. The method is purported to aid weight loss, regulate blood sugar, and enhance heart health. However, it comes with potential risks such as dehydration, nutrient deficiencies, and hormonal disruptions. While it offers autonomy over meal timing and eliminates the need for calorie counting, adherence may be challenging due to the prolonged fasting periods. Alternatives like 16:8

fasting or 5:2 fasting may offer similar benefits with shorter fasting windows, making them more sustainable for some individuals. Ultimately, the suitability of Eat Stop Eat depends on individual preferences, health status, and goals.

## 3. Warrior Diet

The Warrior Diet is an intermittent fasting plan that mimics the eating pattern of ancient warriors, focusing on a 20-hour fasting window followed by a 4-hour eating window each day. Created by Ori Hofmekler, a former member of the Israeli Special Forces, the diet aims to promote weight loss and enhance the body's "survival instincts." However, it's important to note that Hofmekler is not a healthcare provider or registered dietitian nutritionist, and the Warrior Diet has not been extensively studied for its efficacy or health effects.

**The Warrior Diet consists of three phases, each lasting one week:**

**a. Phase One (Detox Week):** During the initial phase, you consume small portions of foods such as broth, hard-boiled eggs, raw vegetables and fruits, yogurt, cottage cheese, and vegetable juices throughout the 20-hour fasting period. During the 4-hour eating window, you're advised to eat a salad with oil and vinegar, along with plant-based foods like vegetables, beans, and whole grains.

**b. Phase Two:** In the second week, you continue to consume the same foods during the fasting period but increase your intake of fats, including nuts, animal protein, and cooked vegetables, during the eating window.

**c. Phase Three:** During the third week, you cycle between high-carb and low-carb days within the 4-hour eating window, incorporating one or two days of each type of eating pattern over the week.

After completing the three phases, you can repeat the process as desired, focusing on a high-protein, low-carb diet, and avoiding grains and processed foods.

While there haven't been specific studies on the Warrior Diet, research on intermittent fasting in general suggests potential benefits such as weight loss, improved blood sugar and insulin levels, cholesterol control, and reduced inflammation. However, the evidence is inconclusive, and more research is needed to fully understand the effects of intermittent fasting on health.

Despite the potential benefits, the Warrior Diet comes with risks and challenges. Nutritional deficiencies can occur due to restricted eating, leading to issues such as fatigue and weakened immunity. Rapid weight loss may also result in adverse effects like abnormal menstrual bleeding, constipation, and gallstones.

Moreover, extreme fasting can be harmful to certain groups of people, including children, individuals with chronic health conditions, pregnant or breastfeeding individuals, and those who take medications that require food. Exercising during fasting hours can increase the risk of dizziness or fainting, posing a safety concern.

## 4. Time Restricted Eating

Time-restricted eating, also known as time-restricted fasting, is a popular approach to dietary patterns that involves restricting the period during which food is consumed while fasting for the remaining portion of the day. One common method of time-restricted eating is the 16/8 or 14/10 method, where individuals fast for 16 or 14 hours respectively, and consume all their meals within an 8 or 10-hour window.

This approach is appealing to many individuals due to its simplicity and flexibility. Since most people naturally fast while they sleep, extending the fasting period until later in the day is relatively easy. For example, with the 16/8 method, one might skip breakfast and delay their first meal until lunchtime, thereby compressing their eating window to 8 hours. Similarly, with the 14/10 method, individuals might delay breakfast slightly further into the morning and conclude their last meal earlier in the evening.

The 16/8 method typically involves eating between the hours of 10 a.m. and 6 p.m., while the 14/10 method involves eating between 9 a.m. and 7 p.m. These eating windows can be adjusted according to individual preferences and lifestyles, making it a versatile option for many people.

One of the key benefits of time-restricted eating is its convenience and adaptability. It can be repeated daily, or done once or twice a week, depending on personal preferences and goals. However, it may take some time to find the right eating and fasting windows that work best for each individual, especially for those who are very active or tend to wake up hungry for breakfast.

It's important to note that while time-restricted eating doesn't necessarily restrict the types of foods consumed, it emphasizes the timing of meals. However, nutritionists often recommend that the majority of calories be consumed earlier in the day before it gets dark out. This is because people tend to choose more calorie-dense, low-nutrient foods at night, and consuming calories earlier in the day allows for better blood sugar regulation and energy utilization throughout the waking hours.

**5. 5:2 Fasting**

The 5:2 fasting method, also known as the twice-a-week method, is a popular approach to intermittent fasting that involves capping calorie intake at 500 for two non-consecutive days of the week while maintaining a regular, healthy diet on the remaining five days. This method offers a structured yet flexible way to incorporate intermittent fasting into one's lifestyle, allowing for both calorie restriction and normal eating patterns throughout the week.

On fasting days, individuals typically consume a 200-calorie meal and a 300-calorie meal, totaling 500 calories for the entire day. It's important to focus on consuming high-fiber and high-protein foods during these meals to help promote satiety and keep calorie intake low. Examples of foods that are commonly consumed during fasting days include lean proteins, vegetables, fruits, whole grains, and legumes.

One of the key advantages of the 5:2 fasting method is its flexibility in choosing fasting days. Individuals can select any two non-consecutive days of the week as their fasting days, such as Tuesdays and Thursdays, as long as there is a non-fasting day between them. This flexibility allows individuals to tailor their fasting schedule to their personal preferences and lifestyle commitments.

It's important to note that on non-fasting days, individuals should continue to eat the same amount of food they normally would, without overcompensating for the reduced calorie intake on fasting days. By maintaining a balanced and healthy diet on non-fasting days, individuals can ensure that they are meeting their nutritional needs and promoting overall health and well-being.

The 5:2 diet is based on the principle of calorie restriction for two days of the week while allowing for normal eating patterns on the remaining days. This approach has gained popularity due to its simplicity and effectiveness for weight management and overall health.

## Timing and Duration Tips

Timing and duration are crucial aspects of intermittent fasting, influencing its effectiveness and suitability for individual lifestyles.

**1. Choose the Right Fasting Window:** Intermittent fasting involves alternating periods of fasting and eating. The fasting window refers to the period during which no calories are consumed, while the eating window is the designated time for consuming meals. Common fasting windows include 16/8 (16 hours fasting, 8-hour eating window), 18/6, 20/4, or even longer fasting periods like 24 hours.

**2. Experiment with Different Eating Patterns:** There's no one-size-fits-all approach to intermittent fasting. Experiment with various eating patterns to find what works best for you. Some people prefer skipping breakfast and eating from noon to 8 p.m. (16/8 method), while others might find it easier to skip dinner instead.

**3. Consider Lifestyle and Schedule:** Choose a fasting schedule that aligns with your lifestyle and daily routine. If you have a busy morning schedule, fasting until lunchtime might be more manageable. Alternatively, if you prefer to have breakfast with your family, consider adjusting your eating window accordingly.

**4. Start Slowly and Gradually Increase Fasting Duration:** If you're new to intermittent fasting, start with shorter fasting durations and gradually increase them as your body adapts. Begin with a 12-hour fasting window overnight and gradually extend it to 14, 16, or more hours over time.

**5. Stay Hydrated During Fasting Periods**: It's essential to stay hydrated, especially during fasting periods. Drink plenty of water, herbal tea, or black coffee to help curb hunger and maintain hydration levels. Avoid sugary beverages or those with added calories, as they can break your fast.

**6. Listen to Your Body:** Pay attention to your body's hunger cues and energy levels during fasting periods. If you feel excessively hungry or fatigued, it's okay to adjust your fasting schedule or break your fast early. Intermittent fasting should not cause undue stress or discomfort.

**7. Be Consistent:** Consistency is key to seeing results with intermittent fasting. Stick to your chosen fasting schedule as much as possible, even on weekends or holidays. Consistency helps regulate hormones, optimize metabolic function, and promote overall health benefits.

**8. Combine with Balanced Nutrition:** Intermittent fasting works best when combined with a balanced diet rich in whole foods. Focus on nutrient-dense meals during your eating window, including plenty of fruits, vegetables, lean proteins, whole grains, and healthy fats. Avoid processed foods, excessive sugars, and refined carbohydrates.

**9. Monitor Progress and Adjust as Needed:** Keep track of your progress, including changes in weight, energy levels, and overall well-being. If you're not seeing the desired results or experiencing adverse effects, consider adjusting your fasting schedule or seeking guidance from a healthcare professional or nutrition expert.

**10. Be Patient and Persistent:** Like any dietary strategy, intermittent fasting requires patience and persistence to see long-term benefits. Stick with it, stay committed to your fasting schedule, and trust the process. Results may take time, but consistent efforts can lead to improved health and wellness over time. ccc ccc)

By following these timing and duration tips, you can customize your intermittent fasting approach to suit your lifestyle, preferences, and health goals effectively. Remember to prioritize balance, consistency, and overall well-being while incorporating intermittent fasting into your routine

## Balancing Nutritional Needs for Optimal Results

Balancing nutritional needs for optimal results in intermittent fasting involves ensuring that your body receives essential nutrients while adhering to fasting protocols. It is important for seniors to:

**1. Meet Macro and Micronutrient Requirements:** Intermittent fasting should not compromise your intake of essential macronutrients (carbohydrates, proteins, and fats) and micronutrients (vitamins and minerals). Focus on consuming a variety of nutrient-dense foods during your eating window to meet your body's needs.

**2. Prioritize Whole Foods:** Emphasize whole, minimally processed foods that provide a broad spectrum of nutrients. Include plenty of fruits, vegetables, whole grains, lean proteins, and healthy fats in your meals to ensure adequate nutrient intake.

**3. Optimize Protein Intake:** Protein is crucial for muscle repair, satiety, and overall health. Aim to include a source of lean protein in each meal to support muscle maintenance and repair, especially during fasting periods.

**4. Choose Complex Carbohydrates:** Opt for complex carbohydrates, such as whole grains, legumes, and starchy vegetables, over refined carbohydrates. Complex carbs provide sustained energy and are rich in fiber, vitamins, and minerals.

**5. Include Healthy Fats**: Incorporate sources of healthy fats, such as avocados, nuts, seeds, olive oil, and fatty fish, into your meals to support brain function, hormone production, and nutrient absorption.

**6. Manage Hydration:** Stay hydrated throughout the day, especially during fasting periods, by drinking water, herbal tea, or other calorie-free beverages. Adequate hydration is essential for overall health and helps curb hunger during fasting.

**7. Time Meals Strategically:** Plan your meals to coincide with your fasting and eating windows, ensuring that you consume essential nutrients when your body needs them most. Consider timing high-protein meals or post-workout nutrition during your eating window to support muscle recovery and growth.

**8. Consider Supplements:** In some cases, supplementation may be necessary to address specific nutrient deficiencies or support overall health during intermittent fasting. Consult with a healthcare professional or registered dietitian to determine if supplements are appropriate for you.

**9. Monitor Portion Sizes:** Be mindful of portion sizes and avoid overeating during your eating window. Practice mindful eating techniques, such as chewing slowly and paying attention to hunger and fullness cues, to prevent excessive calorie consumption.

**10. Listen to Your Body:** Pay attention to how your body responds to intermittent fasting and adjust your dietary choices accordingly. If you experience fatigue, weakness, or other adverse effects, it may indicate a need for more balanced nutrition or a modification of your fasting protocol.

By prioritizing balanced nutrition and mindful eating habits, you can support optimal health and performance while practicing intermittent fasting. Remember that individual nutritional needs may vary, so it's essential to listen to your body and make adjustments as needed to achieve sustainable results.

# Chapter Four

# Recipes for Vitality

Having a meal plan simplifies the process of eating healthily during the eating window. It involves setting aside time to plan meals for the week, creating a shopping list, and preparing meals in advance.

A well-rounded IF meal plan includes lean proteins, fruits, vegetables, carbohydrates, and healthy fats. These components provide essential nutrients, support satiety, and aid in muscle maintenance or building.

**Best Foods for Breaking a Fast:**

**Lean Proteins:** Chicken, pork, beef, beans, legumes, dairy, eggs, fish, shellfish, and tofu.

**Fruits:** Colorful fruits like apples, berries, cherries, peaches, plums, and melons for vitamins, antioxidants, and                                                                                    fiber.

**Vegetables**: Nutrient-rich options such as carrots, broccoli, tomatoes, cauliflower, green beans, kale, spinach, leafy greens, and cabbage.

**Carbohydrates**: Essential for energy and include potatoes, sweet potatoes, oats, rice, quinoa, and whole grains.

**Healthy Fats:** Avocados, nuts, seeds, coconut/MCT oil, butter/ghee, egg yolks, salmon, sardines, olive oil, and avocado oil for nutrient absorption.

**Foods to Avoid:** Processed foods, sugary snacks, candies, sweetened drinks, alcoholic beverages, sugary cereals, and sweetened coffees or teas should be minimized to maintain a healthy eating style.

**Nutrient-Rich Meal Plans**

**Breakfast Recipes**

1. Avocado Toast with Poached Eggs

2. Greek Yogurt Parfait with Berries and Granola

3. Overnight Oats with Banana and Almond Milk

4. Smoothie Bowl with Spinach, Banana, and Chia Seeds

5. Scrambled Eggs with Spinach and Mushrooms

6. Chia Seed Pudding with Coconut Milk and Fresh Fruit

7. Whole Grain Waffles with Fresh Berries and Yogurt

8. Green Smoothie with Spinach, Avocado, and Banana

9. Cottage Cheese with Fresh Fruit and Cinnamon

10. Peanut Butter Banana Toast on Whole whole-grain bread

**Lunch Recipes**

1. Grilled Chicken Salad with Mixed Greens and Balsamic Vinaigrette

2. Quinoa and Black Bean Bowl with Roasted Vegetables

3. Lentil Soup with Whole Grain Bread

4. Grilled Salmon with Brown Rice and Steamed Broccoli

5. Turkey and Avocado Wrap with Mixed Greens

6. Veggie Stir-Fry with Tofu and Brown Rice

7. Chicken and Quinoa Bowl with Roasted Vegetables

8. Whole Grain Pita with Hummus, Cucumber, and Tomato

9. Spinach and Feta Stuffed Chicken Breast with Brown Rice

10. Vegetable and Bean Chili with Whole Grain Crackers

**Dinner Recipes**

1. Grilled Chicken with Roasted Vegetables and Quinoa

2. Baked Salmon with Sweet Potato and Green Beans

3. Vegetable Stir-Fry with Tofu and Brown Rice

4. Lentil and Vegetable Curry with Brown Rice

5. Grilled Turkey Burger on a Whole Grain Bun

6. Chicken and Vegetable Skewers with Quinoa

7. Spinach and Feta Stuffed Chicken Breast with Brown Rice

8. Vegetable and Bean Chili with Whole Grain Crackers

9. Grilled Shrimp with Zucchini Noodles and Cherry Tomatoes

10. Roasted Chicken with Root Vegetables and Quinoa

A 7-day meal plan offers variety and includes recipes such as breakfast salads, mini quiches, and Mediterranean chicken bowls. These recipes are nutritious, flavorful, and suitable for intermittent fasting.

**Day 1:**

**Breakfast (Breaking the Fast)**

- Scrambled eggs with spinach and tomatoes:
1. Wash and chop spinach and tomatoes.
2. Whisk eggs in a bowl.
3. Cook eggs with spinach and tomatoes in a non-stick skillet until set.

**Whole grain toast:**

Toast whole grain bread slices.

**Sliced avocado:**

Slice ripe avocado.

**Lunch**

- **Grilled chicken salad with mixed greens, cucumbers, bell peppers, and a vinaigrette dressing:**
1. Grill chicken breasts seasoned with salt and pepper until cooked through.
2. Prepare mixed greens, cucumbers, and bell peppers for the salad.
3. Prepare vinaigrette dressing.
- Quinoa salad with chickpeas, diced vegetables, and a lemon-tahini dressing:
1. Cook quinoa according to package instructions.
2. Mix quinoa with chickpeas, diced vegetables, and lemon-tahini dressing.

**Dinner**

**Baked salmon with dill and lemon:**

1. Preheat oven to 375°F (190°C).
2. Season salmon fillets with dill, lemon juice, salt, and pepper.
3. Bake salmon for 12-15 minutes until cooked through.

- **Steamed asparagus:**

Trim asparagus spears and steam until tender.

**Roasted sweet potatoes:**

1. Wash and dice sweet potatoes.
2. Toss sweet potatoes with olive oil, salt, and pepper.
3. Roast in the oven at 400°F (200°C) for 25-30 minutes until golden brown.

**Day 2:**

**Breakfast**

**Greek yogurt with mixed berries and a drizzle of honey:**

- Mix Greek yogurt with mixed berries and drizzle with honey.

**Whole grain oatmeal with cinnamon and sliced almonds:**

- Cook whole-grain oatmeal according to package instructions.
- Sprinkle with cinnamon and sliced almonds.

**Lunch**

**Lentil soup with vegetables**

- Cook lentil soup with diced vegetables and seasoning.

**Whole grain roll:**

- Serve with whole grain rolls.

**Side salad with mixed greens, carrots, and balsamic vinaigrette:**

- Prepare mixed greens, carrots, and balsamic vinaigrette.

**Dinner**

**Turkey meatballs with marinara sauce:**

- Prepare turkey meatballs and simmer in marinara sauce.

**Zucchini noodles:**

1. Spiralize zucchini into noodles.
2. Sautee in a skillet with olive oil, garlic, salt, and pepper.

**Steamed broccoli:**

- Steam broccoli florets until tender.

**Day 3:**

**Breakfast**

**Whole grain pancakes with blueberries:**

- Prepare whole grain pancake batter and cook pancakes on a skillet.
- Top with fresh blueberries.

**Greek yogurt topping with walnuts and honey:**

- Serve Greek yogurt with crushed walnuts and a drizzle of honey.

**Lunch**

**Grilled vegetable wrap with hummus in a whole wheat tortilla:**

- Grill mixed vegetables and wrap in a whole wheat tortilla with hummus.

**Side of fruit salad:**

- Prepare a fruit salad with your choice of fruits.

**Dinner**

**Baked chicken breast with rosemary and garlic:**

- Marinate chicken breasts with rosemary, garlic, olive oil, salt, and pepper.
- Bake in the oven until cooked through.

**Quinoa pilaf with mushrooms and peas:**

Cook quinoa with sautéed mushrooms and peas.

**Steamed green beans:**

Steam green beans until tender.

**Day 4:**

**Breakfast**

**Vegetable omelet with mushrooms, onions, and bell peppers:**

1. Sautee mushrooms, onions, and bell peppers in a skillet.
2. Pour beaten eggs over the vegetables and cook until set.

**Whole grain toast with almond butter:**

Toast whole grain bread and spread almond butter on top.

**Lunch**

**Tuna salad lettuce wraps with diced celery and carrots:**

- Mix tuna with diced celery and carrots.
- Wrap in lettuce leaves.

**Whole grain crackers:**

Serve with whole-grain crackers.

**Dinner**

**Stir-fried tofu with mixed vegetables in a ginger-soy sauce:**

Stir-fry tofu and mixed vegetables in a ginger-soy sauce

**Brown rice:**

Cook brown rice according to package instructions.

**Day 5:**

**Breakfast**

**Smoothie with spinach, banana, berries, Greek yogurt, and almond milk:**

Blend spinach, banana, berries, Greek yogurt, and almond milk until smooth.

**Whole grain toast with avocado:**

Toast whole grain bread and top with sliced avocado.

**Lunch**

**Minestrone with whole grain crackers:**

Prepare a minestrone with your favorite vegetables and beans.

**Mixed green salad with feta cheese, olives, and balsamic vinaigrette:**

Toss mixed greens with feta cheese, olives, and balsamic vinaigrette.

**Dinner**

**Grilled shrimp skewers with lemon and garlic:**

1. Marinate shrimp in lemon juice, garlic, olive oil, salt, and pepper.
2. Grill until cooked through.

**Quinoa salad with roasted vegetables:**

Prepare quinoa salad with roasted vegetables of your choice.

**Day 6:**

**Breakfast**

**Cottage cheese with sliced peaches and a sprinkle of cinnamon:**

Serve cottage cheese with sliced peaches and a sprinkle of cinnamon.

**Whole grain toast with avocado:**

Toast whole grain bread and top with mashed avocado.

**Lunch**

**Chicken Caesar salad with romaine lettuce, grilled chicken, Parmesan cheese, and Caesar dressing:**

Prepare Caesar salad with romaine lettuce, grilled chicken, Parmesan cheese, and Caesar dressing.

**Whole grain roll:**

Serve with a whole-grain roll.

**Dinner**

**Baked cod with herbs and lemon:**

- Season cod fillets with herbs and lemon.
- Bake until cooked through.

**Steamed broccoli:**

Steam broccoli florets until tender.

**Quinoa with diced tomatoes and basil:**

Prepare quinoa with diced tomatoes and fresh basil.

**Day 7:**

**Breakfast**

**Veggie and cheese omelette:**

Make a veggie and cheese omelet with your choice of vegetables and cheese.

**Whole grain toast with almond butter:**

Toast whole grain bread and spread almond butter on top.

**Lunch**

**Lentil and vegetable stew:**

Prepare lentil and vegetable stew with your choice of vegetables and seasoning.

**Whole grain roll:**

Serve with a whole-grain roll.

**Dinner**

**Grilled steak with roasted potatoes and green beans:**

- Grill steak to the desired doneness.
- Roast potatoes until golden brown.
- Steam green beans until tender.

**Side salad with mixed greens and balsamic vinaigrette:**

Toss mixed greens with balsamic vinaigrette.

**General Tips:**

1. Prepare ingredients in advance to streamline meal preparation throughout the week.
2. Store leftovers in airtight containers for easy reheating and meal assembly.

3. Adjust portion sizes based on individual preferences and dietary needs.

4. Stay hydrated by drinking plenty of water throughout the day.

5. Enjoy the meals mindfully during the eating window, savoring the flavors and nourishing your body.

## Culinary Delights Supporting Senior Wellness

As a senior, it's essential to prioritize nutrient-dense meals while fasting to maintain energy and support overall health. Healthy cooking techniques can help preserve nutrients and make cooking easier, even on fasting days.

**Simple Cooking Methods:**

1. **Roasting**: Roasting is a great way to cook vegetables, meats, and fish without added oils. It helps retain nutrients and brings out natural flavors. Simply season with herbs and spices, and roast in the oven until tender.

2. **Grilling**: Grilling is a low-fat cooking method that adds a smoky flavor to foods. Use a non-stick grill or grill pan to prevent sticking and retain nutrients.

3. **Sautéing**: Sautéing is a quick and easy way to cook vegetables, meats, and fish with minimal oil. Use a non-stick pan and cook over medium heat until tender.

**Tips for Cooking with Ease:**

1. **One-Pot Meals:** One-pot meals are a great way to cook multiple ingredients in one pot, reducing cleanup and preserving nutrients. Try making soups, stews, or skillet meals.

2. **Slow Cooker Recipes:** Slow cookers are perfect for fasting seniors, as they allow for hands-off cooking and retain nutrients. Simply add ingredients and cook on low for 6-8 hours.

3. **Batch Cooking:** Batch cooking involves preparing large quantities of food and reheating as needed. This saves time and reduces food waste.

4. **Prep in Advance**: Chop vegetables, marinate meats, and prep ingredients in advance to make cooking easier and faster.

5. **Use Herbs and Spices:** Instead of salt and sugar, use herbs and spices to add flavor to your meals. This reduces sodium and added sugars.

6. **Keep it Simple:** Focus on simple recipes with fewer ingredients to reduce stress and cooking time.

7. **Use Healthy Oils:** Use healthy oils like olive, avocado, or grapeseed oil for cooking and dressing.

## Meal Planning and Grocery Shopping Tips for Fasting Seniors

As a senior, meal planning and grocery shopping can be challenging, especially when fasting. However, with some simple strategies, you can plan healthy meals and snacks, shop on a budget, and navigate the grocery store with ease.

**Meal Planning Tips:**

1. Plan Ahead: Plan your meals and snacks for the week, considering your fasting schedule and dietary needs.

2. Keep it Simple: Focus on simple, one-pot meals and snacks that are easy to prepare and require minimal ingredients.

3. Include Electrolyte-Rich Foods: Incorporate electrolyte-rich foods like bananas, avocados, and leafy greens into your meals to maintain electrolyte balance.

4. Prep in Advance: Chop vegetables, marinate meats, and prep ingredients in advance to make cooking easier and faster.

5. Consider Your Nutrient Needs: Ensure your meals and snacks provide essential nutrients like protein, healthy fats, and complex carbohydrates.

**Grocery Shopping Tips:**

1. Make a List: Create a shopping list based on your meal plan to avoid impulse buys and stay on budget.

2. Shop the Perimeter: Focus on the grocery store's perimeter, where fresh produce, meats, and dairy products are typically located.

3. Buy in Bulk: Purchase non-perishable items like nuts, seeds, and canned goods in bulk to save money.

4. Opt for Affordable Protein Sources: Choose affordable protein sources like beans, lentils, and eggs.

5. Use Coupons and Sales: Take advantage of coupons, sales, and promotions to reduce your grocery bill.

6. Shop at Local Markets: Consider shopping at local farmers' markets or discount grocery stores for fresh produce and affordable prices.

7. Avoid Processed Foods: Limit processed foods, which are often high in sodium, added sugars, and unhealthy fats.

8. Read Labels: Read food labels to ensure you're getting the nutrients you need and avoiding unwanted ingredients.

# Chapter Five

# Fitness and Strength

## Incorporating Exercise for Enhanced Results

Exercise during intermittent fasting may increase fat burning, but it's also conceivable that you won't have as much energy and won't be able to work out as hard. Paying attention to your body is crucial.

**Benefits and drawbacks of working out when fasting**

Before deciding to work out while fasting, weigh the benefits and drawbacks of doing so if you're trying intermittent fasting (IF) or are fasting for other reasons but still want to get your workouts in.

Exercise during a fast has been found to impact muscle biochemistry and metabolism, which is related to insulin sensitivity and stable blood sugar regulation.

Eating and exercising right away, before digestion or absorption, is also supported by research. For those who have metabolic syndrome or type 2 diabetes, this is very crucial.

One benefit of fasting is that you will probably burn more fat since your glycogen, or stored carbohydrates, will be reduced.

Does burning more fat seem like a good thing? There's a drawback to the fasted cardio trend before you hop on it. If you exercise while fasting, your body may begin metabolizing muscle to use protein as fuel. Additionally, "you're more likely to run into a wall, which means you won't have as much energy to work out or perform as well."

According to Priya Khorana, EdD, a nutrition educator at Columbia University, long-term exercise and intermittent fasting are not the best options. "Your metabolism may eventually slow down as a result of your body depleting itself of calories and energy," she continues.

Should you work out while you're fasting?

- You might burn fat at a higher rate.

- An extended period of fasting may cause your metabolism to slow down.

- Exercise may not be as effective for you.

- You might not be able to gain muscle; instead, you might only be able to retain it.

**Performing well in a workout while fasting**

There are a few things you can do to maximize your workout if you're determined to pursue intermittent fasting (IF) while keeping up your fitness regimen.

1. Consider the timing When trying to maximize the effectiveness of your fasting exercise, registered dietitian Christopher Shuff suggests three things to think about whether to work out before, during, or after the fuelling window. A widely used IF technique is the 16:8 protocol. The idea is to eat everything within an 8-hour window for fueling and then refrain from eating for 16 hours.

"Those who perform well when exercising on an empty stomach should work out before the window, while those who dislike working out on an empty stomach and wish to maximize post-workout nutrition should work out during the window," he says.

The optimum option, according to Shuff, is during both performance and recovery. He continues, "Those who prefer to work out after fueling but are unable to do so during the eating window should use the after-the-window period."

2. Select the training style according to your macros. Lynda Lippin, a master pilates instructor and certified personal trainer, emphasizes the significance of monitoring your macronutrient intake the day before and the day after an exercise session. Strength training, for instance, usually calls for higher carbohydrate intake the day of the session, whereas cardio and HIIT (high-intensity interval training) can be done on a day with fewer carbs.

**3. Consume the correct foods to maintain or gain muscle after working out.**

The greatest way to combine IF with exercise is to schedule your workouts for when your nutrition is at its highest, right before or right after meals. "And if you lift a lot of weight, it's critical for your body to have protein to help with regeneration after the workout." Within 30 minutes of finishing your workout, Amengual advises consuming 20 grams of protein and some carbohydrates in addition to strength training.

**How can you work out while fasting without risk?**

The safety of a weight loss or fitness program's long-term sustainability determines its success. You must remain in the safe zone if your ultimate objective while using IF is to reduce body fat and maintain your current level of fitness. Here are some expert pointers to assist you in doing that.

**1. Have a meal shortly before engaging in a moderate-to-intense workout.**

Here's when the timing of meals becomes important. It's important to eat right before or after a moderate- to high-intensity workout. In this manner, your body has some glycogen reserves that it can use to power your exercise.

2. **Remain hydrated.**

Keep in mind that fasting does not imply dehydration. He advises increasing your water intake during the fast. Maintain your electrolyte levels. Coconut water is a great low-calorie hydration option, "It tastes pretty good, replenishes electrolytes, and is low in calories,". Sports drinks like Gatorade contain a lot of sugar, so try not to consume them in excess.

3. **Maintain a moderate level of intensity and duration.** Take a rest if you exert too much energy and start to feel lightheaded or dizzy. It's crucial to pay attention to your body.

4. **Think about the kind of fast**

Sticking to low-intensity exercises like strolling, restorative yoga, and light Pilates if you're on a 24-hour intermittent fast. Sticking to a specific kind of exercise isn't as important if you're following the 16:8 fast, though, as the majority of the 16-hour fasting window is spent in the evening, sleeping, and early morning.

5. Pay attention to your body.

The most crucial piece of advice to follow when working out during IF is to pay attention to your body.

"If you start to feel weak or dizzy, chances are you're dehydrated or you have low blood sugar." If so, she advises choosing a carbohydrate-electrolyte drink right away and then having a well-balanced lunch afterward.

Some people may find that exercising and intermittent fasting work well together, but others may find that exercising in any way during a fast is uncomfortable for them.

## Building Strength in the Golden Years

**How to strengthen and coordinate yourself better**

It turns out that a decrease in physical activity is one of the main factors contributing to the loss of strength and coordination that comes with aging. There is a misconception in our culture that says getting older doesn't mean you have to exercise less. The reverse is true! Regular exercise becomes increasingly necessary as you age. You may even want to increase the amount of time you spend exercising to offset hormonal changes in your body and other uncontrollable factors. The good news is that people of all ages can benefit from strength and coordination workouts. (Take note, though, that as you get older, you might need to exercise more caution to avoid being hurt. Ask your doctor or a physical therapist what kinds of workouts are appropriate for you if you're unsure.)

**Regardless of Age difference, you can undertake the following exercises to strengthen and coordinate your body:**

1. Engage in cardiovascular activities for at least thirty minutes, five days a week, such as jogging, biking, swimming, or brisk walking.

2. Engage in at least two hours a week of strength, balance, and flexibility-enhancing activities, such as yoga, tai chi, Pilates, and isometric weightlifting.

3. Play sports like basketball, tennis, and golf that you'd like to get better at.

4. Make the most of the guidance and instruction provided by coaches, trainers, and teachers to enhance your fitness abilities.

5. Consult your physician to manage conditions that may hinder your capacity to exercise, such as movement disorders like Parkinson's, cataracts, and other eye issues, as well as orthopedic injuries.

6. A Mediterranean diet rich in fish, olive oil, avocados, fruits, vegetables, nuts, legumes, whole grains, and chicken will nourish your mind and muscles. Eat other foods in moderation.

7. Get enough rest so that you can sharpen your talents during the night.

# Chapter Six

## Navigating Challenges

### Overcoming Potential Obstacles

Attempting intermittent fasting (IF) can be a life-changing event and has several health benefits. But, it has its own set of difficulties, just like any big lifestyle adjustment. We're going to look at five typical concerns that a lot of our community members have when they first start IF and offer doable fixes to assist you get over these obstacles with confidence.

**1. Managing cravings and understanding hunger**

Dealing with hunger and craves during fasting periods is one of the initial obstacles with IF. When your body gets used to a new eating pattern, it's normal to have hungry sensations. However, if you eat well, these spells should pass quickly.

First, give your body time to adjust by progressively extending your fasting window. Second, when you're within your eating window, be sure you're eating the correct items. Consuming whole foods that are high in fiber, and healthy fats, and your recommended daily intake of 60g of protein will help you feel filled for longer periods and be prepared for fasting. We can assist you in organizing your meals so that you are well-nourished and able to fend off hunger. Last but not least, drink plenty of water, herbal teas, and black coffee—all of which are suitable for fasting and can help reduce hunger and thirst.

## 2. Balancing family dinners with social meals

Strict dietary restrictions can make it difficult to participate in social events and family dinners.

One potential solution is to organize your fasting schedule to coincide with social events whenever feasible. For instance, if you regularly enjoy a family meal together in the evening, consider delaying your eating window until later in the day to accommodate that. During your fasting period, if you are invited to a meal, choose a fasting-friendly option to eat if you are following a 5:2 diet, or concentrate on the social aspect of the meal rather than the food if you are following time-restricted eating (TRE). In most cases, a meal can be modified to fit your needs on the menu. As an alternative, give yourself special events a break in your IF schedule.

## 3. Preserving vitality

Some people may have low energy periods, particularly in the early stages of IF.

**Solution:** To maintain energy levels, make sure your eating windows include balanced meals full of minerals, high-quality protein, and healthy fats. A Mediterranean-style diet, which includes all the essential macro and micronutrients to keep you running, even during a fast, is naturally high in energy and can help minimize symptoms of exhaustion. Furthermore, pay attention to your body and modify your fasting window as needed. Try shifting your fasting window to an earlier time of day, for instance, if you find that skipping breakfast makes you feel lethargic. Last but not least, maintaining adequate hydration can also support maintaining mental and physical energy. Black coffee has no calories and can be drunk during a fast if you need a little push, even though you shouldn't rely on caffeine to keep you going.

## 4. Handling emotional eating

Eating is much more than just satisfying hunger for a lot of people. For people who turn to food as a coping mechanism for stress or other emotions, it can be difficult.

**Solution:** Create different coping strategies to deal with emotional stress, such as working out, practicing meditation, or taking up a hobby. Managing emotional eating can be aided by being aware of emotional triggers, and interacting with others can ensure that you are not struggling alone. Mindfulness training has been demonstrated to help prevent emotional eating and support weight reduction efforts.

## 5. Motivation and consistency

It can be challenging to maintain consistency and motivation, particularly when weight loss seems to be plateauing or progressing slowly.

The answer is to track your progress and set reasonable targets. Reward yourself for modest accomplishments to stay motivated. Recognize that there are strategies to overcome weight loss plateaus and that they are very normal. Joining a group of like-minded IF practitioners can also offer encouragement and support.

**Adapting Fasting to Individual Health Considerations**

Adapting intermittent fasting to individual health considerations, such as type 2 diabetes, heart disease, obesity, and other health conditions, requires careful planning and consultation with healthcare professionals. Here are some considerations for adapting intermittent fasting to specific health needs:

**Type 2 Diabetes:**

- Individuals with type 2 diabetes should approach intermittent fasting with caution and under the guidance of a healthcare provider. Fasting can affect blood glucose levels and insulin sensitivity, which may require adjustments to diabetes medication or insulin dosage.
- Consider shorter fasting periods or modified fasting protocols, such as time-restricted eating (e.g., 14/10 method), to minimize the risk of hypoglycemia (low blood sugar) and stabilize blood glucose levels.
- Monitor blood sugar levels closely during fasting periods and be prepared to break the fast if blood sugar drops too low. Stay hydrated and prioritize nutrient-dense foods during eating windows to support overall health and blood sugar control.

**Heart Disease:**

- Individuals with heart disease or cardiovascular risk factors should focus on heart-healthy eating patterns during both fasting and eating periods. Emphasize whole foods, such as fruits, vegetables, lean proteins, and healthy fats, while limiting processed foods, added sugars, and saturated fats.

- Consider intermittent fasting protocols that prioritize cardiovascular health, such as the Mediterranean diet combined with time-restricted eating. This approach emphasizes plant-based foods, fish, olive oil, and moderate wine consumption, which have been associated with reduced risk of heart disease.

- Monitor blood pressure, cholesterol levels, and other cardiovascular risk factors regularly, and consult with a healthcare provider to ensure that intermittent fasting is safe and appropriate for your heart health.

**Obesity:**

- Intermittent fasting can be a useful tool for weight management and obesity treatment when combined with a balanced diet and regular physical activity. However, it's essential to approach fasting with a focus on long-term sustainability and overall health rather than quick fixes or extreme restrictions.

- Choose intermittent fasting protocols that align with personal preferences, lifestyle, and health goals. Experiment with different fasting schedules, such as alternate day fasting, the 5:2 method, or time-restricted eating, to find what works best for you.

- Pay attention to hunger cues, energy levels, and mood during fasting periods, and adjust your fasting protocol as needed to ensure that it supports your well-being and adherence to healthy eating habits.

**Other Health Conditions:**

- Individuals with other health conditions, such as gastrointestinal disorders, mental health disorders, or autoimmune conditions, should approach intermittent fasting with caution and consider potential impacts on symptoms and overall health.

- Consult with healthcare professionals, including primary care physicians, registered dietitians, and specialists, to determine the safety and appropriateness of intermittent fasting for your specific health needs.

- Be mindful of medication timing and potential interactions with fasting, especially for medications that require food intake. Work with healthcare providers to adjust medication schedules or dosages as needed to accommodate fasting periods.

- Monitor symptoms and overall well-being closely during fasting periods, and be prepared to modify or discontinue fasting if it negatively affects health or exacerbates underlying conditions.

In summary, adapting intermittent fasting to individual health considerations requires a personalized approach that considers medical history, current health status, and individual needs and preferences. Consulting with healthcare professionals and prioritizing overall health and well-being is essential for safely incorporating intermittent fasting into a health-conscious lifestyle.

# Chapter Seven

## Mindful Living

### Incorporating Mindfulness Practices

The practice of fasting has a long history and rich cultural heritage. Its roots can be found thousands of years ago in many different religions and cultures, where it was frequently practiced as a means of self-control and spiritual reflection. For example, Muslims fast from sunrise to sunset during the holy month of Ramadan as a means of engaging in spiritual introspection, cultivating gratitude for nourishment, and practicing mindfulness. A key idea in Buddhism is mindful awareness, and one way to practice mindfulness is by fasting.

Moving forward to the present, mindful approaches can also be used with intermittent fasting. The technique of purposefully going without food for predetermined amounts of time, together with developing awareness of one's own bodily and emotional reactions to the fast, is known as "mindful fasting." It entails identifying and monitoring sensations of hunger and fullness, the mind's reaction to not eating, and the body's physiological responses, much like traditional mindfulness practices. To promote a deeper awareness of one's connection with food and eating patterns, mindful fasting emphasizes being fully present and engaged during the fasting experience rather than just the act of not eating.

Both mindful eating and mindful fasting can support you as you advance in your quest for better health. You may learn when to start and finish eating a meal as well as when to break or start a fast by paying attention to your hunger and fullness indicators. You can even enhance your perception of taste and smell throughout a fast by practicing mindfulness, which will help you enter your Fast Breaker with a greater awareness of and appreciation for the meal you're going to consume. Consequently, this can enhance your mindful eating experience and raise the likelihood that you will reap the numerous advantages of eating intuitively.

**Tips on mindful Eating and mindful Fasting**

In addition to increasing self-awareness, combining mindful eating and mindful fasting encourages better eating practices, self-control, and a more balanced relationship with food.

The following tips will assist you in incorporating mindful fasting and mindful eating into your daily nutritional regimen.

## 1. Use the Scale of Hunger to Fullness to Determine When to Break a Fast

In mindful eating practices, a hunger-fullness scale is a self-awareness tool that people can use to recognize and respond to their body's natural hunger and satiety cues. It usually has a range of 1 to 10, where 1 denotes intense hunger, 10 severe fullness or pain from overeating, and the medium range denotes a comfortable sensation of contentment and fullness.

The hunger-fullness scale might help you determine when you've had enough food when you're eating. When you feel satisfied but not overly full, you should ideally end your meal when you are between a 7 and an 8 on the scale. You can use this tool to support your fasting practice as well. (Prolonged fasting excluded) Ideally, you would break your fast when your hunger reaches roughly a 3. This may lead to a different length of the fasting period for the day a shorter or longer fast is acceptable. But before you break that fast, consider utilizing this as an opportunity to gain a deeper knowledge of what hunger feels like and the messages your body is sending you. You might discover that a small amount of hunger is more acceptable than you previously believed, or you might acquire an understanding of when your body needs to be fed and for how long.

**2) Prepare a Mindful Meal for Your Fast Break**

It has been demonstrated that eating mindfully that is, consuming meals when you are at ease, in the moment, and not distracted produces health and longevity benefits, such as enhanced metabolic health and weight loss. Combining this routine with your Fast Breaker can foster gratitude for eating and assist in determining how much your body truly requires at any one time. A more decadent eating window has the potential to counteract some of the benefits of fasting; still, a thoughtful Fast Breaker may lessen that risk.

According to studies, eating without interruption reduced the number of calories taken later on in addition to the number of calories consumed during the meal or snack. Therefore, if and when you want to break your fast, do so in a focused and distraction-free manner. It will be easier for you to concentrate on feeding your body, which will eventually improve your health. Additionally, the first bite after breaking your fast usually tastes the greatest, so savor it while it lasts!

**3) If necessary, break your fast.**

We frequently break our fasts out of habit, although our bodies might not truly require it at that particular time. For example, having breakfast is a normal household custom that many of us practice as soon as we wake up! But, some of us who practice mindfulness while fasting may discover that breakfast is more of an ingrained eating habit than a true need for energy and nourishment.

We can adjust the duration of our daily fasts based on what our bodies are telling us at any given time. For instance, your body can require nutrients sooner the next day if you mistakenly underrate or had a strenuous workout the day before. Conversely, you can also experience a day in which you feel happy, alert, and full of energy. You may choose to extend your fast that day until your body requires food, even if you met your usual fasting objective.

## 4) Develop a Greater Appreciation for Food via Mindfulness

Fasting has the special power to improve our appreciation of food and change the way we think about it. When we purposefully skip meals for a set amount of time, we develop a keen awareness of our bodies' natural hunger signals and what it feels like to eat when we do. Our relationship with food can change as a result of this increased awareness, as we begin to see it more as a necessary source of nourishment rather than just something to be enjoyed. We can discover that we are engaging in mindful eating if we find ourselves enjoying every bite and focusing on the flavor, texture, and perfume of our food.

We might choose more consciously, choosing nutrient-dense foods that nourish our bodies, as a result of our heightened awareness.

In conclusion, while eating and fasting may seem like straightforward ideas, making conscious choices about them will help you avoid the diet trap (which has been proven to be ineffective) and achieve steady short- and long-term benefits. Instead of being strict, the idea is to get more in tune with your body and mind to improve your relationship with yourself, gain a better understanding of how food affects your general health, and become more self-aware.

**Enhancing Mental Clarity and Focus**

Intermittent fasting can have both positive and negative effects on mental clarity and focus, depending on various factors such as the duration and type of fasting, individual health status, and overall lifestyle. Here's an overview of how intermittent fasting may impact mental health and practical tips for enhancing mental clarity and focus while fasting:

**Positive Effects on Mental Health:**

Short-term fasting periods may enhance mental clarity and focus for some individuals, This is because fasting can lead to changes in neurotransmitter levels, alterations in energy metabolism, and activation of cellular repair processes like autophagy.

Fasting triggers the production of ketones, which serve as an alternative energy source for the brain, potentially enhancing cognitive function and protecting against neurodegenerative diseases.

Fasting promotes the release of brain-derived neurotrophic factor (BDNF), a protein important for learning, memory, and mood regulation, which may contribute to improved cognitive performance and resilience to stress and depression

**Negative Effects on Mental Health:**

Prolonged or extreme fasting may contribute to mood disturbances and cognitive impairments. Research suggests that certain fasting practices could increase symptoms of depression, anxiety, anger, irritability, and stress, particularly if not properly managed.

Fasting may not be suitable for everyone, especially individuals with certain medical conditions like diabetes or a history of eating disorders. Pregnant women, children, and those experiencing an acute mental health crisis should avoid fasting due to potential risks.

# Chapter Eight

## Success Stories

### Real-Life Testimonials of Seniors Embracing Ageless Energy

@Shelby I was diagnosed with diabetes at 28. I still remember it was my first sugar test and my fasting sugar level was whooping 456. It's been two years, quit medicine immediately after 6 months of diagnosis, and now fasting sugar ranges between 70-90. Intermittent and keto have helped me a lot and it does work!

@David Did it for 3 months, and it works. Not only helped with weight loss but also made my mind relaxed and light. It made me focus on studying more than I did. Loved the energy and vibes I got when I fasted.

@Danny Hey everyone this works...like she said if you do it correctly it will benefit you! Starting Sept I was 205 because of quarantine. Now I'm at 175! Eat healthy lots of nutrients & plenty of water & most of all...exercise! Be productive with your body every day if you can ☐ good luck to everyone god bless you ☐☐

@Rose I'm a type 1 diabetic and I've been doing the 16:8 fast for a week now and my blood sugar levels are EXPONENTIALLY better!

@Frankie I'm 44 and reached a point in my life where I want everything that I put into my mouth to benefit me nutritionally. I have a cheat meal on the weekend but Monday- Friday it's fasting & eating healthy. It is hard but you have to be disciplined because the long-term benefits are completely worth it

@Angelique Intermittent fasting is the only reason I went from 200 to 120 lbs. I didn't go hard on exercise or choosing healthy meals. I ate whatever I wanted during my one meal a day.

@Edward I noticed that when I skip breakfast I have a lot of energy and don't get too tired quickly. I sometimes sleep very late and wake feeling energetic. This is great honestly. I eat around noon or sometimes 1 PM. I drink water and coffee in the morning.

@Cristabel Been on IF for 6 months, lost 22 kgs / 48 lbs. Started at 108 kgs / 238 lbs and now at 86 / 190. Aside from a week of being a grumpy ogre, I found the shift into ketosis quite simple. Plus I know so much more now, it's easier to eat more nutrition than junk. Walking or cycling daily, to burn 350-500 calories. A couple of months ago decided to start pushups, now at 20x5 sets a day

# Chapter Nine

# FAQs

**1. How does intermittent fasting operate and what does it entail?**

The intermittent fasting (IF) diet involves eating for extended periods interspersed with deliberate fasting or extremely low-calorie intake. It is thought by researchers that IF causes a metabolic shift in which fat is used instead of glucose as the main energy source. Additionally, it may benefit the circadian cycles of growth hormone and insulin secretion as well as gut biology. It can enhance weight regulation and energy metabolism in several ways.

**2. Why does blood sugar rise during a fast?**

When someone fasts, their blood glucose levels decrease. This results in an increase in glucagon production by the pancreas, a hormone that keeps blood sugar levels from dropping too low. This is made possible by glucagon's capacity to cause the liver to break down glycogen, or stored glucose, and release glucose back into the bloodstream. Moreover, glucagon increases blood glucose retention by blocking the liver's ability to absorb and store glucose. The body recognizes when more glucagon is not needed thanks to a feedback system. When all is well, the body will produce insulin to offset the elevated glucose levels by transferring glucose from the blood into the cells.

On the other hand, the body either uses insulin ineffectively or the pancreas does not produce enough of it in a diabetic. Consequently, elevated glucose levels remain in the blood.

**3. Does the evidence point to the improvement of human health parameters by IF?**

Animals have been used in IF studies more often than humans. Although there is encouraging data to suggest improvements in people's health, many of the clinical trials conducted to date have used very brief interventions spread out over several months. Nearly all IF studies produced some weight loss, ranging from 2.5% to 9.9%, and related fat mass decrease, according to a 2018 review article. It may be a better weight loss strategy than other diets and eating habits, however, there isn't much evidence to support this claim.

Blood pressure may also benefit from the application of an IF diet. In one study, 1,422 participants were examined for a year while adhering to a fasting regimen. The subjects' blood pressure decreased in both the systolic and diastolic ranges. Researchers discovered that IF offered metabolic and cardiovascular benefits, including a reduction in total cholesterol and low-density lipoprotein (LDL) cholesterol, in another study involving adult males. Researchers have found that calorie restriction improves insulin resistance. Insulin levels fall and insulin sensitivity rises during a fasting period. Blood sugar levels are improved as a result of these modifications while fasting and shortly after eating.

**4. Regarding individuals with type 2 diabetes, what are the potential hazards associated with IF?**

IF can cause a range of side effects. Feeling lightheaded, vomiting, sleeplessness, Falls related to syncope, migraine-related headaches, a vulnerability that restricts day-to-day activity, and extreme hunger cravings. An individual's chance of encountering numerous adverse consequences could be elevated by a chronic illness like diabetes. When taking insulin or other drugs like sulfonylureas, patients with type 2 diabetes are also susceptible to hypoglycemia. With other diabetes drugs, this risk is reduced, but it is still present. Another danger is dehydration. Dehydration can happen if a person doesn't drink enough fluids, even though they can drink calorie-free beverages on "fasting days." Following dehydration, hypotension may occur. People may need to cut back on or stop taking some drugs entirely on fasting days. These include diuretics, antihypertensive, and SGLT-2 inhibitors, a class of diabetes drugs that can cause dehydration. But it's crucial to always see a doctor before stopping or adjusting the dosage of a drug.

### 5. Is type 2 diabetes reversible with IF?

Three guys were able to use IF to reverse their insulin resistance in a single small case series. This made it possible for individuals to control their blood sugar levels even after they stopped using insulin. They also lost weight, saw a decrease in their waist circumference, and saw a drop in their hemoglobin A1c levels. It would be more correct to state that these people are in remission of their diabetes, though, as relapse is a possibility.

Researchers also randomly assigned individuals to one of two groups in the Diabetes Remission Clinical Trial (DiRECT) weight management or pharmaceutical therapy. It was shown that 46% of the individuals in the group that managed their weight achieved diabetic remission. Nevertheless, there has been little research done thus far, necessitating more investigation.

## 6. Is there a reason a person with type 2 diabetes shouldn't attempt intermittent fasting?

IF may exacerbate symptoms in individuals with labile diabetes, also known as brittle diabetes by others, and in those whose blood sugar levels are difficult to control. Little study has been done on how IF affects certain groups of people, like those who are nursing or pregnant.

Additionally, those who are more susceptible to adverse effects like hypoglycemia, dehydration, and hypotension ought to stay away from IF. This group comprises elderly individuals, those with weakened immune systems, and those who have previously experienced dementia or traumatic brain injury. In addition, intentional fasting might exacerbate the difficulties faced by those suffering from eating disorders.

## 7. How many type 2 diabetics safely practice intermittent fasting?

Before beginning IF, a diabetic should speak with their physician to make sure it's safe for them. To lower their chance of hypoglycemia, a person will also require their doctor's advice on changing the amounts and timing of their prescriptions. People attempting intermittent fasting (IF) should check their blood sugar more often, ideally every 2-4 hours, especially in the beginning.

When a person has hypoglycemia, they should break their fast right away and take glucose pills or gels, which contain 15 grams of carbs, to raise their blood sugar. They ought to see a physician before resuming the fast. To lower the danger of dehydration and hypotension during the fasting period, it's also critical to consume more fluids. Certain diabetes drugs, diuretics, and antihypertensives may need to be stopped or their dosage reduced, according to a doctor's advice. On non-fasting days, people should have a balanced diet and stay away from processed, fatty, and sugary foods. By doing this, they will ensure that the benefits of the fasting days are maintained.

## 8. Can individuals with type 2 diabetes benefit from any of the IF's dietary recommendations?

The science of intermittent fasting has several diet implications. A circadian rhythm governs the changes in insulin sensitivity, which diminishes over the day and into the night. Consequently, eating a meal at night is linked to increased insulin and glucose levels. Restricting eating hours to earlier in the day might help increase metabolism and promote weight loss. For instance, choose an 8-hour window between 7 a.m. and 3 p.m. or even 10 a.m. and 6 p.m. Additionally, people ought to make an effort to refrain from eating and snacking right before bed. Avoiding between-meal snacks will speed up the metabolic transition from using glucose to fat for energy.

A balanced diet is also essential, so people should steer clear of processed carbohydrates and sugars and instead prioritize eating whole grains, fruits, vegetables, lean meat, and healthy fats. Selecting an eating plan that an individual can stick to over time is maybe the most crucial component.

# Conclusion

# Embracing a Life of Vitality and Strength

As you conclude your journey through "Intermittent Fasting for Seniors: An Essential Handbook for Vitality and Strength for Ageless Energy," it's essential to reflect on the key concepts you've learned and consider your next steps toward embracing a life of vitality and strength.

## Recap of Key Concepts:

Throughout this handbook, you've discovered the transformative power of intermittent fasting for seniors. You've learned how intermittent fasting can support vitality and strength as you age by promoting cellular repair, improving metabolic health, and enhancing cognitive function. By incorporating intermittent fasting into your lifestyle, you have the opportunity to optimize your overall well-being and enjoy ageless energy.

**Key concepts covered in this handbook include:**

1. Understanding the science behind intermittent fasting and its effects on aging.

2. Exploring different intermittent fasting protocols and finding the approach that suits your preferences and health goals.

3. Learning how to adapt intermittent fasting to individual health considerations, such as managing chronic conditions or supporting heart health.

4. Discovering practical tips and strategies for safely implementing intermittent fasting into your daily routine, including meal planning, hydration, and monitoring your body's signals.

**Next Steps on Your Ageless Energy Journey:**

As you embark on your journey toward vitality and strength, consider the following next steps to continue your                                          progress:


1. Reflect on your experiences with intermittent fasting and how it has impacted your energy levels, overall health, and quality of life.

2. Consult with healthcare professionals, including your primary care physician and registered dietitian, to discuss your intermittent fasting practice and ensure it aligns with your individual health needs and goals.

3. Continue to educate yourself on the latest research and developments in intermittent fasting and aging to stay informed and empowered in your wellness journey.

4. Explore complementary strategies for enhancing vitality and strength, such as regular physical activity, stress management techniques, and social engagement.

5. Embrace a mindset of lifelong learning and growth, recognizing that age is just a number and that you have the power to cultivate ageless energy at any stage of life.

In closing, remember that "Intermittent Fasting for Seniors" is not just a handbook—it's a roadmap to a life filled with vitality, strength, and ageless energy. By embracing the principles of intermittent fasting and prioritizing your well-being, you have the opportunity to live your best life and thrive as you age. Here's to a future filled with health, happiness, and endless possibilities!